Vedda Blood Sugar Remedy

Robert Parisi

CONTENTS

I. INTRODUCTION

Welcome to "Vedda Blood Sugar Remedy: Vedda-Based Remedy and HIIT Training Protocol"! This book is going to provide readers with a deep insight into one of the most popular global lethal diseases: diabetes, including both type I and type II diabetes.

As a matter of fact, the ultimate solution to diabetes does not lie in the most recent technology, but in the ancient therapies of our ancestors, especially the dietary strategies of a group of native inhabitants living in the deep forests of Sri Lanka.

Therefore, I have written this book to provide you with the foundation knowledge on how to fight against this terrible condition using lifestyle patterns from the past, combined with the famous modern HIIT training program.

Before digging into the main contents of this book, I must emphasize that if you have already been diagnosed with high blood pressure, then the first thing you should do is consult your doctor for drugs and related issues. Make sure that you discuss anything you are going to do with your doctor to promote better results.

By strictly following the real-life strategies laid out in this book, you will be able to dramatically reduce the development of diabetes. Having analyzed the potential harms resulting in high blood sugar, this book indicates an entire process of cutting down on your blood sugar level.

Every chapter of this guidebook is compiled and written based on the real-life case studies and experience from me, as well as other prestigious health specialists all over the world.

Last but not least, do not forget to enjoy your own journey when flipping through the pages of this book. When you finish this book, you will sooner or later realize that eliminating diabetes from your life is challenging yet worth trying. Thank you and good luck!

II. CHAPTER I: WHAT IS DIABETES?

What is diabetes?

Nowadays, because of the unhealthy eating habits and lifestyle, the number of people who have suffered from diabetes keeps increasing over time. According to statistics shown by the International Diabetes Federation, more than 387 million cases of diabetes are recorded. Moreover, by the end of 2035, that figure will have reached 592 million. More notably, it is also reported that there is one person who dies every seven seconds because of diabetes.

It sounds alarming, isn't it? So, what actually is diabetes?

Diabetes happens when the body's ability to produce and respond to the hormone insulin is weakened. When your body does not have the sufficient amount of insulin, it cannot regulate the level of glucose in the blood. That leads to the imbalanced concentration of glucose, which is the primary form of sugar. Our body needs the energy to function every day and glucose is the body's key source of energy. It is extracted from what we eat in our daily life.

There are different types of diabetes, including type I diabetes, type II diabetes, pre-diabetes, gestational diabetes and latent autoimmune diabetes. We will discuss in more detail in the next part.

Types of diabetes

Basically, diabetes type I and II are the two most common ones. So, let's get to know them better!

Type I diabetes is also called idiopathic or immune mediated diabetes. It usually occurs in the group of young people. In this diabetes type, the beta cells, which exists in the Islets of Langerhans areas, are destroyed. Since these cells are insulin producer, without them the pancreas cannot generate any insulin. Therefore, the body is unable to convert glucose into energy. Instead, the sugar from food remains in your blood or passes all the way to the urine.

You know you have type I diabetes when the following situation appears:

- Losing weight uncontrollably

- Feeling fatigue more often

- Having blurry vision

- Having headaches

- Feeling weak

- Getting skin infection

- Being Dizzy

- Passing excessive urine

- Being extremely thirsty

Type II diabetes is more common than Type I, and it often occurs in the old group of people (normally, over 45 years old). It makes up for approximately 85 percent of all diabetes patients. With this type II, the pancreas does not produce adequate insulin, or the insulin made does not work properly. Hence, there is also an excess amount of sugar left in your blood. While other cells, which are in need for glucose, cannot access to it. Consequently, the body feels weak, lethargic, and lack of energy. Additionally, over time the pancreas of people with type II diabetes will lose the capacity to produce insulin. As a result, the situation will get worse and worse. That even leads to fatal cases.

You know you have type I diabetes when the following symptoms appear:

- Excessive urination

- excessive thirst

- lethargy

- Slow healing cuts

- Unexplainable hunger

- Leg cramps

- Blurry vision

- Gradual weight gain

- Mood swings

- Skin infections

Except those diabetes types, there are also other ones such as Gestational Diabetes Mellitus (GDM), Pre-diabetes and Latent autoimmune diabetes of adults (LADA.).

Gestational Diabetes Mellitus is identical to Type II in some extents. It exists mostly in pregnancies and might seriously harm the mother health if it is not treated properly. Fortunately, people can simply cure GDM by using thorough and full medical treatment with the consultancy of experts during the pregnant period.

Pre-diabetes happens when the level of sugar in one's blood is excessive but not high enough to be considered as type II diabetes. People who develop type II, often undergo pre-diabetes for an extended period.

LADA is a form of diabetes type I, in which even though the presence of islet antibodies at diagnosis of diabetes, the development time is rather slow. People sometimes are mistaken it with type II as its symptoms, and those at the beginning of type II share some similar characteristics.

Cause of diabetes

Scientists have not found out the exact cause of both types. With the type II, many say that your family history, age, and ethnic background does impact the chance of developing diabetes. That means you are likely to grow diabetes if you inherit the genes from your parents or grandparents who already have the disease.

To be specific, if you have any of the following issues, the likelihood to acquire type II diabetes is higher:

- High blood pressure

- Over weight

- Lack of physical activity

- Improper diet

- Your family have the history of suffering from diabetes

- You are 45 years old or above and have one of the above conditions

- You are above 55 years old

How diabetes impacts the health

Diabetic ketoacidosis is one of the most common complications of the type I diabetes. At this stage, you will experience a disorder of metabolism manifested in vomiting, abdominal pain, nausea, breathing problems.

Kussmaul breathing is the deep breathing that takes place during diabetic ketoacidosis. There is also an issue related to the odor of acetone in the breath.

You might also experience the **Hyperosmolar non-ketonic** condition during diabetes. It often appears in type II diabetes due to dehydration.

Above all, **Blood vessels,** however; is the most sophisticated and dangerous complication. There is up to 75% cases of deaths caused by diabetes related to coronary artery situation. Because of the harms in blood vessels, it leads to the damage your nerves, kidneys, and eyes.

The disadvantages of conventional medication

It is common that people with diabetes get prescription medication from the doctor to treat their disease. However, many studies and experiments are revealing that the most effective medication is a good dietary habit with frequent exercise. The reason is the causes of this disease are mostly from an unhealthy eating habit and lifestyle. Moreover, the medication used for patients with type II diabetes very often causes side effects.

There is no permanent cure for type II diabetes. The most prevalent drug for this disease is Metformin, which is proved to be able to regulate the level of sugar in your blood. Although this medication can benefit the patients by synthetic insulin, there are significant side effects that might happen. People taking this drug can experience some health issues such as dizziness, digestive problems, hormonal disruption, and sinus Infection. Additionally, research in 2010 revealed that Metformin could considerably reduce the amount of B12 in your body. As a result, that deficit heightens the risk of heart attacks and other related cardiovascular diseases.

Other common drugs for diabetes like Sulfonylureas, Biguanides, Alpha-glucosidase Inhibitors, Thiazolidinediones, Meglitinides, and DPP-4 Inhibitors can also make you prone to many serious problems because of their side effects. It not to mention, those medications do not eliminate the disease.

In essence, the primary cause of type II diabetes is the unhealthy lifestyle and an imbalanced diet. Thus, the best cure for this disease is to adopt a good way of living with a proper eating habit and exercise on a regular basis.

So, what should you do to prevent and treat this life-threatening illness? The answer lies beyond my two next chapters. I have been researching this topic for a long time since my cousin suffers from it. I have been reading numerous of books, articles, blogs. In the following chapter, I will be presenting to you all valuable knowledge that I have learned, including my experience with curing my cousin's disease.

III. CHAPTER II: EVERYTHING YOU NEED TO KNOW ABOUT VEDDA BLOOD SUGAR REMEDY

Everyone who is finding the way to fight against diabetes might come across the name "Vedda blood sugar remedy" once a twice time. This is one of the newest and most effective methods to treat people with diabetes, especially with type II.

In this chapter, I will tell you everything about the magical treatment of the Vedda people. Keep reading until the end; you might find some helpful inputs.

Vedda Origin

To fully understand how Vedda originally started, let's have a closer look at this intimidating culture, so we will be able to understand the secret dietary strategies, along with lifestyle habits that make them stand out as the population that has never had any diabetes patient recorded.

As a matter of fact, the Vedda are local settlers based in Sri Lanka, and they have been renowned for being forest occupants who are the one of the late generations of the Neolithic ancestors. It is reported that the Vedda people are generally divided into three different groups; namely, Anuradhapura Veddas, Bintenne Veddas and Coast Veddas.

These groups are in several geographical areas across Sri Lanka and seem to have no contact with one another. The estimated population in Sri Lanka is 6,600 people, accounting for a small minority of the Sri Lankan population (approximately 20 million people).

The primary Veddan preoccupation is hunting, with men being the major source of labor. In addition to using primitive weapons like arrow and bow to hunt wild animals, toxic plants are also utilized to kill the targeted preys. Regarding the main language, Vedda people's mother tongue is reported to be a unique one, not to mention that they also have an interesting worship system.

The Vedda Dietary Habits

Vedda people are popular for having a meat-rich diet. The major sources of meat which are utilized as food are rabbit, tortoise, wild board, turtle, brown monkey, venison and monitor lizard. Fish is also a common food choice. Gona perume is a delicacy which the Vedda enjoys savoring. To be specific, gona perume is defined as a kind of sausage that consists of alternating meat and fat layers.

One of the most favorite dishes among the Vedda population is goya-telperume, which includes monitor lizard's tail combined with fat. Additionally, dried meat which is preserved in honey is another delicacy which the Vedda considers as their favorite dish.

Overall Impression

The Vedda people have been living in the Sri Lankan jungles for thousands of years, building up simple lifestyles surrounded by fishing, growing crops and hunting. In general, their diet contains a significant amount of protein which is stored in these kinds of meats: rabbit, tortoise, wild boar, venison, turtle, monitor lizard, and brown monkey.

The Vedda's dietary habits also consist of eating various fruits and vegetables that are rich in fiber and vitamins such as maize, gourds, yams, melons and coconut. It has come as no surprise that the way the Vedda eat is almost like what Western health specialists argue as a diabetes-free lifestyle.

Regarding type II diabetes, it is vital that your blood sugar levels are balanced. Luckily, there are multiple foods which able to promote that positive result, especially those that contain huge amounts of fiber, protein and healthy fat.

The combination of these three substances can help you maintain your blood sugar at a healthy level. On the other hand, the two most dangerous factors that mess with your well-being state are carbs and sugar. Although your body requires decent carbohydrate consumption to survive, the necessary amount is very tiny.

Another wise piece of advice is to consume foods which are high in the mineral chromium, with the typical example being broccoli. Scientists have also announced that magnesium can do wonders for your blood sugar conditions, which is basically the reason why grass-fed beef, along with other types of seeds, vegetables and nuts are strong weapons to fight against diabetes.

The Western medical sector has concluded that fiber is an essential element when it comes to curing diabetes. Coconut oil is also an ideal candidate as it can help you burn additional fat and get your blood sugar levels under control through its healing properties.

Proper protein intake is also an important requirement. Salmon is always voted as a good protein alternative, as well as organic chicken, turkey and grass-fed beef.

Powerful Components for Diabetes Elimination

Coconut

I strongly believe that coconuts are a special present that nature has given human beings. It is one of the key staple sources utilized to keep your body vigorous and healthy that people have eaten for centuries. In the case of the Vedda people, they have great interests in coconuts, and they tend to add its pulp or milk into almost anything they eat.

Due to its magical ability to improve longevity and general wellness, coconuts have been gradually appreciated by the Western science. Nevertheless, most people are yet to recognize that coconut is a perfect ingredient in terms of being diabetes' enemy.

Besides, coconut oil can protect your body from being infected with bacteria, viruses, thyroid cancer, and heart-related problems. Another plus point for this healthful substance is that it helps maintain the beauty of your skin, as well as burn extra fat off your body.

Particularly, coconut fiber has been found to promote a blood-sugar-lowering effect. The amount of carbohydrates consumed are converted into blood sugar, which is scientifically called glucose. Pre-diabetics and diabetics are advised to eat foods which are low in glycemic index. Foods which rank high in the glycemic index are identified as potential culprits for developing diabetes.

Your body realizes that an increase in blood sugar is a terrible sign, so it will immediately start pumping insulin into your blood vessels to bring things back to normal. Since coconut oil can inhibit the absorption process of sugars to your body, your blood sugar will be kept at a safe level. Moreover, coconut oil is also able to enhance your body's blood circulation.

In a nutshell, coconut oil is extremely beneficial to your diabetes condition compared to other types of oil products. Indeed, coconut oil is the best option to reverse the negative effects of diabetes, as well as maintain the balance of your blood sugar.

In case you eat a meal that happens to elevate your blood sugar to a dangerous level, a few tablespoons of coconut oil is a good instant solution. Your blood sugar is expected to return to a normal level within half an hour.

Cinnamon

Cinnamon is usually regarded as a newly found herb utilized to add flavors to your dishes. Also, it has a magic factor which helps your body prevent your blood sugar levels from overreacting to foods. Gradually, your body's sensitive reaction to insulin will be dramatically enhanced. To put it another way, your body will only have to release a small amount of insulin to eliminate the excess sugar from your blood.

Basically, those who develop diabetes will not be able to react to insulin the way normal people do. This condition is called insulin resistance – a situation in which your body rejects insulin. As a matter of fact, insulin is essential to our body because it functions as a kind of chaperone to remove sugar from your blood and get it into the cells within the body.

If insulin cannot make it into your body's cells, the blood sugar inside will not change, leading to several serious consequences for your health. Specifically, high blood sugar can destroy blood vessels located around the eyes, causing blindness. Likewise, the nerves within your limbs can also be negatively affected, thus causing the malfunction of a lot of different body parts.

Therefore, cinnamon enables your body to sensitively respond to insulin efficiently. According to a study published in December 2003 involving sixty type II diabetes patients, those who were treated with cinnamon experienced a remarkable decrease of 18 to 29% in the amount of blood glucose compared to those who were prescribed with a placebo.

Neem

Not only is the Neem tree common in Sri Lanka's forest zones, but it is also very popular with the native Indian sub-continent citizens. It is believed that the leaves, bark, and leaves of these trees can cure 40 diseases, so it has been used for a couple thousand years by the Vedda people.

The most essential ingredients contained in Neem trees are antioxidants and cancer-fighting components that can destroy gum disease and infections. Neem has been reported to lower insulin requirements by approximately 50% without having to change the levels of blood glucose just by stimulating the pancreas' beta-cells to release insulin.

Ginger

The ginger's root has been applied to deal with digestive issues and enhance general wellness for many centuries. Although the results might not be very clear, it can help you reduce the risks of diabetes. Over the recent years, the medical sector is becoming more and more interested in the healing properties of ginger. Even though researchers are yet to figure out why ginger can improve diabetes, they have identified some healthful ingredients like paradols, zingerone and shogaols.

These mentioned substances all can reverse the terrible impacts of diabetes. Another scientific study suggests that both human beings and animals can obtain tremendous health benefits from ginger for arthritis, cardiovascular health, cancer and diabetes.

Essential Anti-Diabetes Minerals

Chromium

Chromium used to be known as GTF, which is the short form of Glucose Tolerance Factor. This substance is a mixture of d-nicotinic acid, glutathione and chromium 3, functioning like a type of insulin. Hence, it plays the role of a transportation means transferring from the outside of the cell to its inside. So, the rapid development of diabetes might also be attributed to chromium deficiency.

Insulin resistance is one of the uncomfortable results of type II diabetes, which means that the human's body cannot react to insulin properly. More than ten studies documented that glucose supplementation can enhance glucose uptake. When its usage is combined with biotin, it will promote powerful effects not for your glucose uptake, but also for the health of your liver.

Chromium can regulate the blood glucose levels, as well as lowering the fat storage to assist in your weight loss process. Besides, chromium can transform the sugar in your body into the necessary energy, thus cutting down on your blood sugar, cholesterol and insulin levels. So, what you need to do to increase the daily chromium consumption is to eat more oysters, turkey, onions, seafood, broccoli, salmon, liver, and eggs.

Magnesium

In fact, magnesium deficiency results in a sharp increase in the intracellular calcium, thus causing insulin resistance. Moreover, insulin resistance may lead a huge amount of insulin being removed from your body through urination. European countries consider diabetes as a magnesium-wasting illness.

Proper magnesium consumption can help your body's muscles constrict again hypertension. Some common magnesium-rich foods are nuts, green leafy, nut, seeds and legumes.

Vanadium

Vanadium is also an important trace mineral which triggers glucose transport and oxidation, not to mention that it takes part in the production of glycogen in your muscles and liver. Not only does it prevent the glucose production from fat, but it can also prevent glucose absorption from the gut. These mentioned factors play key roles in the body's internal glucose metabolism.

Besides, vanadium is also regarded as a credible alternative for insulin since it can improve the sensitivity of insulin receptors in the cell membrane. Other beneficial effects of vanadium on the human body are obstructing the production of cholesterol, reversing cancerous properties and so on. In contrast, a lack of vanadium is likely to result in an elevated mortality rate, slow growth, hypoglycemia, diabetes, insulin resistant and infertility.

The Powerful D

As a matter of fact, over 90% of Native Americans develop Vitamin D deficiency. Specifically, Vitamin D deficiency's ramifications can be classified into two different groups, including short-term implications and long-term implications.

Particularly, some of the most typical symptoms of short-term implications are fibromyalgia, depression and muscle aches. Nevertheless, it is the long-term implications that are extremely dangerous, as they can lead to osteoporosis, cardiovascular disease, cancer and diabetes.

Therefore, a rise in Vitamin D consumption allows your body to fight against type II diabetes by reducing the risk of insulin resistance, as well as decreases the danger of endothelial dysfunction. Moreover, most obese people tend to be lacking in Vitamin D, and they are the most vulnerable individuals to type II diabetes. Thus, Vitamin D deficiency detection is one of the top priorities when it comes to treating both diabetes and obesity.

Habitual Factors of the Vedda

There are some major principles that we can pick up from the Vedda lifestyle and adapt to our circumstances.

Movement

The Vedda people lead a completely proactive lifestyle. To be more specific, men participate in fishing and hunting, whereas the female counterparts indulge in growing crops and cooking. Overall, they rarely sit in a corner doing nothing. So, the first piece of advice for all of us is to exercise.

Healthy Habits

Besides, the Vedda people do not use cigarettes or any other type of tobacco. Additionally, it is reported that there has never been any recorded case of illegal drugs or alcohol usages. The message for us, the modern citizens, is to eliminate unnecessary medications, recreational drugs and smoking.

Stress-free

The Vedda's lives are also calming, peaceful and, of course, stress-free. They never must steer their minds to daily problems like deadlines, traffic jams or mortgage payments. Hence, it is vital that we learn to lower our stress levels.

How to Apply These Principles to Real-Life Situations?

Exercise

Here are ten simple, yet efficient tips that you should keep in mind to keep track of the exercise plan even though there will be times that all you want to do is give up.

1. If your ultimate aim is to possess a healthy body, try to divide that goal into three smaller achievable goals, then note them down like you have already finished them, such as "I lost five pounds in two weeks, and I feel great!" After that, bring that note along with you anywhere you go to remind yourself to keep up with that objective.

2. An effective method to avoid boredom is to alternate the workout schedule on a regular basis. For example, you can vary your detailed program every two months, including different sets of workout exercises and training paces.

3. After sticking with the chair in your office for two hours, stand up and do some push-ups, squats or planks, and you will immediately feel better.

4. Having a small meal every four hours can dramatically enhance your metabolic system, and protein consumption, as well as supply your body with a decent amount of carbohydrates that helps you stay energized throughout the day.

5. A combination of weight training and anaerobic system enables your heart to exercise more efficiently.

6. Practicing HIIT (High Intensity Interval Training) sessions is

another stunning method to keep your body in shape and burn off additional fat. HIIT consists of a series of continuous cardiovascular exercises, including sprinting, rowing or cycling, combined with active rest intervals of about ten seconds.

7. When it comes to the times that you do not feel like doing anything, let alone go to the gym for a hardworking workout session, opt for an only ten-minute exercise on the treadmill.

Stop Smoking

Smoking has been found to be directly associated with 25 lethal diseases, such as stroke, emphysema, heart attack, chronic bronchitis, and cancer. Speaking of smoking, the consequences it causes for your general wellness are even more severe.

Smoking leads to an unbalanced level of blood sugar, as well as prevents your organs' inflammation, not to mention that nicotine is reported to increase the A1-c levels. A1-c is a kind of hemoglobin regarded as an indicator which illustrates how your blood sugar is controlled. On average, smokers have a higher amount of A1-c levels than non-smokers.

Here are some possible solutions to help you kick off this terrible habitual activity.

1. Constantly remind yourself of the healthful benefits you are going to receive once you succeed in eliminating smoking from your life. To be specific, you can make a long list of the advantages of quitting.

2. Conduct a detailed analysis of your smoking patterns such as the situations and times that you are most likely to smoke. This helps you predict future circumstances which can be tempting.

3. Decide a particular date when you will thoroughly get rid of the

habit and mark it on your calendar.

4. Re-organize your surroundings by throwing away anything related to smoking like matches and ashtrays. Additionally, you can also clean off the smell of tobacco on your clothes.

5. Share your smoking-free objective with your friends and acquaintances to ask them for encouraging words.

6. Exercise on a regular basis, and go to places where smoking is not allowed, such as art galleries or museums.

7. Hydrate yourself as much as possible. Besides, it is also important that you eat foods which are low in calories.

Five Quick Tips for Reducing Stress Levels

Exercise

As noted in this book, the advantages of exercise have been discussed, but now we are going to have a closer look at the way exercise lowers your stress levels. In fact, exercise is not only an underused antidepressant, but it is also underrated compared to other methods.

According to many scientific studies, frequent cardiovascular exercise can significantly enhance your concentration and mental alertness, remove stress, as well as improve both general mental and physical health. In fact, after a five-minute session of exercise, your body's ability to produce endorphins has been greatly improved, making you feel more comfortable.

Love Yourself

Approximately 90% of our internal thoughts are controlled by subconscious area of our brains, especially the negative feedbacks we make for ourselves. Therefore, daily confident affirmations allow you to reflect yourself in a more positive way. Sentences such as "I can do this" or "This is what I can achieve" are great starting points.

Sleep Away

When you think your stress level is becoming unbearable, sleep should be the first thing that comes to your mind. Human body needs to have enough sleep to function properly. While we are sleeping, our bodies can repair the malfunctioning tissues, as well as recalibrate hormonal and chemical imbalances.

If you encounter sleeping difficulties, creating a comfortable atmosphere for your room is an ideal option. Some specific solutions are to turn off the lights, adjust the air-conditioner to a cooler temperature, and stay away from electronic devices.

Healthy Eating Patterns

We are more likely to consume the wrong foods when under stressful situations. Instead of the dangerous junk foods, a dietary plan which is rich in protein and fiber, along with a limited amount of carbohydrates enables you to recover from stressful circumstances.

On the other hand, coffee consumption is actually not beneficial for our stress-dealing methods. As a matter of fact, caffeine may slowly destroy our nervous system.

Make a To-Do List

Spending at least 10 minutes before going to bed on planning the detailed schedule of the following day lets you predict and reduce the amount of burden you have currently had. Preparing a thorough agenda for a day also allows you to sleep more peacefully without having to memorize everything when you go out for shopping.

Reduce Alcohol Consumption

Ethanol, or ethyl alcohol, is the primary component contained in alcoholic beverages. Specifically, this substance stems from the sugar or starch's yeast fermentation. Nearly any starchy or sweet food can be transformed into alcohol.

The human body cannot digest alcohol, so 95% of the alcohol consumed is absorbed by the blood vessels starting from the intestine and stomach in less than an hour. The rest of the 5% is removed via the lungs, skin or kidneys, then your liver will start metabolizing alcohol.

How long this process lasts totally depends on the amount of alcohol combined with food. Generally, nevertheless, it takes between three and five hours to totally metabolize an amount of 30 milliliters of alcohol. As alcohol is broken down, toxic byproducts emerge, destroying the normal functions of your liver. As a result, it dramatically increases the risk of inflammation and fatty liver.

Here are some other interesting methods to lower the alcohol intake in your body:

- Get rid of all alcohol in your house

- Become the designated driver

- Opt for mineral water or tea when eating out

- Drink ten glasses of water every day

Body Detox

To maximize the potentials of the Vedda dietary strategies, the first things that you must do is remove the toxins your body has accumulated. And a one-day detox is an optimum choice to do it.

Acid Overload

One severe consequence of the toxins' infestation into your body is that it messes up your pH levels. The balance between an alkaline liquid and an acidic internal environment plays a key role in maintaining our general wellness.

Our bodies function properly when they reach an alkaline state, so when the acidic levels within our bodies' fluids become too high, we make up for it by releasing minerals from muscles, bones, ligaments and so on. That's why involuntary donor organs are extremely vulnerable to illnesses.

So, what we need to do is eliminate acid from the body's systems, which means that we must remove the ingested harmful toxins that we consume through the external atmosphere or foods.

Why Detox?

The principles behind detoxing is to get rid of the toxins inside your body, thus improving our energy, as well as soothing our digestive system. Besides, it can also burn off additional amounts of fat and help you strengthen your physical heath. After all, your body can be stronger to defend itself against harmful bacteria.

Detox 101

"Detox" originally means blood-cleansing, which is carried out by eliminating the impurities from inside the liver where the consumed toxins are processed. Other body parts which are known as detoxifiers are the skin, the lymphatic system, the lungs, the skin and the blood. Nevertheless, these natural detoxing centers might easily be clogged up, inhibiting them from fully functioning.

When to Detox

You may have already known the advantages of detoxing, and it is about time you started planning for doing it. You should conduct careful research in terms of detox regimens to select the most suitable one for your requirements. If you are a beginner, a one-day cleanse may be a good starting point. By applying this session, your body can stay away from the usual pressure and analyze all unnatural foods you must put up with.

Diet Modifications

The first two components you need to remove from your dietary patterns are coffee and alcohol. Junk foods, fried foods and fast foods should also be crossed out. The next ingredients that need to be on the removal list are grains, processed foods, dairy foods, and meat.

In contrast, it is important that you replace junk foods with components that will reinvigorate and cleanse your body. A few great choices are grown fruits, legumes, green vegetables and raw seeds.

Next, I am going to introduce nine simple tips for a successful one-day detox session.

- Choose natural foods

- Opt for a hot lemon juice or a piece of fruit after waking up

- Include salads, fresh vegetables and fruits

- Add organic protein

- Include Celtic salt

- Use herbal tea

- Opt for cold-pressed coconut oil or olive oil

- Use apple cider vinegar to stimulate digestion

- Add seeds and nuts

The 30-Day Blood Sugar Reduction Protocol

Daily Meal Template

Although your food choices can be different from one day to another due to personal preferences, here is a common template which can utilized to determine which kind of foods you should eat for every single meal.

Meal	What to Eat
Breakfast	Shake, 1 egg, Salad, Vegetables
Brunch	Fruit
Lunch	Poultry, Peas, Salmon, Vegetables, Lamb
Afternoon Snack	Fruit
Dinner	Fish, Peas, Salmon, Vegetables, Poultry

Detailed 30-Day Dietary Plan

Day	What to Eat	Necessary Supplements
Day 1	**One-Day Detox:** - 1 tablespoon of apple cider vinegar - 1 tablespoon of lime juice - 1 tablespoon of pure honey - 1/8 teaspoon of turmeric - 1/8 teaspoon of rosemary - 1/8 teaspoon of cayenne pepper **Fresh Fruit**	Ten 8-ounce water glasses
Day 2	- Breakfast: 2 eggs / banana / coconut milk - Lunch: Dry fruit and Mushroom - Dinner: Mushroom and Chicken Stew	• Chromium – 1000 mcg • Magnesium – 400 mg • Vitamin D – 800 IU

Day 3	- Breakfast: Mushroom Omelette - Lunch: Vegetable Soup - Dinner: Pork Stew and Apple Cider Vinegar	• Chromium – 1000 mcg • Magnesium – 400 mg • Vitamin D – 800 IU
Day 4	- Breakfast: Black Beans with Italian Sausage - Lunch: Chiken Wings with Peanut Butter - Dinner: Cranberry Meatballs	• Chromium – 1000 mcg • Magnesium – 400 mg • Vitamin D – 800 IU
Day 5	- Breakfast: Paleo Bread - Lunch: Barbeque Sausages - Dinner: Stuffed Cabbage Rolled Leaves	• Chromium – 1000 mcg • Magnesium – 400 mg • Vitamin D – 800 IU

Day 6	- Breakfast: Coconut Waffles with Almond Flour - Lunch: Honey-Rubbed Pork Wraps - Dinner: Sour and Sweet Pork	• Chromium – 1000 mcg • Magnesium – 400 mg • Vitamin D – 800 IU
Day 7	- Breakfast: Eggs Poached in Avocado - Lunch: Tuna & Salmon Muffins and Lime Sauce - Dinner: Piquant Chicken	• Chromium – 1000 mcg • Magnesium – 400 mg • Vitamin D – 800 IU
Day 8	- Breakfast: Vegetable Soup - Lunch: Barbeque Sausages - Dinner: Turkey Barbeque Wraps	• Chromium – 1000 mcg • Magnesium – 400 mg • Vitamin D – 800 IU

Day 9	- Breakfast: Almonds, Fruit and Coconut Chips - Lunch: Vegetable Soup with Beef - Dinner: Cranberry Meatballs	• Chromium – 1000 mcg • Magnesium – 400 mg • Vitamin D – 800 IU
Day 10	- Breakfast: Devilled Eggs - Lunch: Shrimp & Garlic with Coconut Milk - Dinner: Cranberry Meatballs	• Chromium – 1000 mcg • Magnesium – 400 mg • Vitamin D – 800 IU
Day 11	- Breakfast: Black Beans with Italian Sausages - Lunch: Chicken Wings with Peanut Butter - Dinner: Cranberry Meatballs	• Chromium – 1000 mcg • Magnesium – 400 mg • Vitamin D – 800 IU

Day 12	- Breakfast: Paleo Bread - Lunch: Barbeque Sausages - Dinner: Stuffed Cabbage Rolled Leaves	• Chromium – 1000 mcg • Magnesium – 400 mg • Vitamin D – 800 IU
Day 13	- Breakfast: Coconut Waffles with Almond Flour - Lunch: Honey-Rubbed Pork Wraps - Dinner: Sour and Sweet Pork	• Chromium – 1000 mcg • Magnesium – 400 mg • Vitamin D – 800 IU
Day 14	- Breakfast: Poached Eggs with Avocado - Lunch: Tuna & Salmon Muffins and Lime Sauce - Dinner: Piquant Chicken	• Chromium – 1000 mcg • Magnesium – 400 mg • Vitamin D – 800 IU

Day 15	- Breakfast: Vegetable Soup - Lunch: Barbeque Sausages - Dinner: Turkey Barbeque Wraps	• Chromium – 1000 mcg • Magnesium – 400 mg • Vitamin D – 800 IU
Day 16	- Breakfast: Devilled Eggs - Lunch: Shrimp & Garlic with Coconut Milk - Dinner: Cranberry Meatballs	• Chromium – 1000 mcg • Magnesium – 400 mg • Vitamin D – 800 IU
Day 17	- Breakfast: Mushroom Omelette - Lunch: Vegetable Soup - Dinner: Pork Stew and Apple Cider Vinegar	• Chromium – 1000 mcg • Magnesium – 400 mg • Vitamin D – 800 IU

Day 18	- Breakfast: Black Beans with Italian Sausages - Lunch: Chicken Wings with Peanut Butter - Dinner: Cranberry Meatballs	• Chromium – 1000 mcg • Magnesium – 400 mg • Vitamin D – 800 IU
Day 19	- Breakfast: Coconut Flakes, Raisins and Walnuts - Lunch: Barbeque Sausages - Dinner: Stuffed Cabbage Rolled Leaves	• Chromium – 1000 mcg • Magnesium – 400 mg • Vitamin D – 800 IU
Day 20	- Breakfast: Coconut Waffles with Almond Flour - Lunch: Honey-Rubbed Pork Wraps - Dinner: Sour and Sweet Pork	• Chromium – 1000 mcg • Magnesium – 400 mg • Vitamin D – 800 IU

Day 21	- Breakfast: Poached Eggs with Avocado - Lunch: Tuna & Salmon Muffins and Lime Sauce - Dinner: Piquant Chicken	• Chromium – 1000 mcg • Magnesium – 400 mg • Vitamin D – 800 IU
Day 22	- Breakfast: Vegetable Soup - Lunch: Barbeque Sausages - Dinner: Turkey Barbeque Wraps	• Chromium – 1000 mcg • Magnesium – 400 mg • Vitamin D – 800 IU
Day 23	- Breakfast: Devilled Eggs - Lunch: Shrimp & Garlic with Coconut Milk - Dinner: Cranberry Meatballs	• Chromium – 1000 mcg • Magnesium – 400 mg • Vitamin D – 800 IU

Day 24	- Breakfast: Mushroom Omelette - Lunch: Vegetable Soup - Dinner: Pork Stew and Apple Cider Vinegar	• Chromium – 1000 mcg • Magnesium – 400 mg • Vitamin D – 800 IU
Day 25	- Breakfast: Black Beans with Italian Sausages - Lunch: Chicken Wings with Peanut Butter - Dinner: Cranberry Meatballs	• Chromium – 1000 mcg • Magnesium – 400 mg • Vitamin D – 800 IU
Day 26	- Breakfast: Coconut Flakes, Raisins and Walnuts - Lunch: Barbeque Sausages - Dinner: Stuffed Cabbage Rolled Leaves	• Chromium – 1000 mcg • Magnesium – 400 mg • Vitamin D – 800 IU

Day 27	- Breakfast: Coconut Waffles and Almond Flour - Lunch: Honey-Rubbed Pork Wraps - Dinner: Sour and Sweet Pork	• Chromium – 1000 mcg • Magnesium – 400 mg • Vitamin D – 800 IU
Day 28	- Breakfast: Poached Eggs with Avocado - Lunch: Tuna & Salmon Muffins and Lime Sauce - Dinner: Piquant Chicken	• Chromium – 1000 mcg • Magnesium – 400 mg • Vitamin D – 800 IU
Day 29	- Breakfast: Vegetable Soup - Lunch: Barbeque Sausages - Dinner: Turkey Barbeque Wraps	• Chromium – 1000 mcg • Magnesium – 400 mg • Vitamin D – 800 IU
Day 30	- Breakfast: Devilled Eggs - Lunch: Shrimp & Garlic with Coconut Milk - Dinner: Cranberry Meatballs	• Chromium – 1000 mcg • Magnesium – 400 mg • Vitamin D – 800 IU

Step-by-Step Recipes for the Protocol

Mushroom Omelet

Ingredients:

- 1 cup of chopped mushrooms
- 2 teaspoons of nondairy milk
- ½ cup of egg beaters
- 1 teaspoon of olive oil
- 1 dash of pepper
- 1 dash of salt

Instructions

Stir-fry the mushrooms within olive oil at least four minutes until soft. Mix salt, pepper, milk, and olive oil, with egg substitute. Heat up the skillet for half a minute, then combine the egg mixture with it. Cook for another two minutes until set, then add the mushrooms and stir-fry for two more minutes.

When the omelet is about to be done, turn the plate over and cook the opposite side using a spatula. This dish is served with vegetables.

Black Beans with Italian Sausages

Ingredients

- 12 oz, of chopped Italian sausage
- ½ chopped onion
- ½ cup of black beans
- ½ cup of tomato puree

- 1½ cup of minced green chilies
- 2 basil leaves
- 1 teaspoon of pepper
- ¾ tablespoon of salt
- 1 teaspoon of vegetable oil

Instructions

Sauté the chilies and onions with olive oil for approximately 5 minutes using a crockpot. After that, add the other ingredients, put the lid on, and leave it on for about three hours on slow heat.

Devilled Eggs

Ingredients

- 6 hard-boiled eggs
- ¼ cup of pureed avocado
- 1 dash of black pepper
- 2 teaspoons of vinegar
- 1 dash of salt

Instructions

Break the eggs, then cut them lengthwise into halves. Remove the yolks and put them aside. Mix other ingredients with the yolks until the texture turns smooth. Divide the yolk mixture into equal servings and you're done.

Coconut Flakes with Walnut Raisins

Ingredients

- ¼ cup of walnuts
- ¼ cups of raisins
- ½ cup of sugar-free coconut chips or flakes

Instructions

Combine all the ingredients together within a large bowl, then serve with nondairy milk (optional).

Poached Eggs with Avocado

Ingredients

- 3 avocados
- 3 eggs

Instructions

Poach eggs to your own taste, then put them inside the avocadoes. Sprinkle with pepper and serve.

Vegetable Soup

Ingredients

- Celery
- Yellow squash
- Leeks
- Garlic
- Vegetable broth
- Oregano
- Salt
- Green beans
- Zucchini

- Red peppers
- Onions
- Shredded cabbage
- Basil

Instructions

Cut up, then mix the vegetables using a pot with heated vegetable broth. Wait until it reaches the boiling point, and wait for it to simmer for about 15 minutes. Add oregano, basil and salt for flavor.

Chicken Wings with Peanut Butter

Ingredients

- 5 chicken wings
- 1 teaspoon of salt
- 1 cup of water
- 3 tablespoons of peanut butter
- 1 tablespoon of ground ginger

Instructions

Mix all the ingredients within a cooker and put the lid on. Leave it on the stove for at least five hours until it softens and serve.

Dry Fruit and Mushroom

Ingredients

- ½ cup of button mushrooms
- 2 cups of chopped almonds

- 1 cup of chopped cashews
- 2 cardamom cloves
- 1 chopped onion
- 2 garlic cloves
- 1 teaspoon of salt
- 1 teaspoon of olive oil
- 1 cup of water

Instructions

Sauté the onion and garlic cloves using a slow cooker and wait until the outsides turn brown. After that, mix the remaining ingredients and wait for 6 to 7 more hours.

Barbeque Sausages

Ingredients

- 1 chopped onion
- 12 oz. of smoked sausages
- 2 tablespoons of apple cider vinegar
- ½ teaspoon of paprika powder
- 1 teaspoon of salt
- 1 teaspoon of cayenne pepper
- ½ cup of water
- 1 teaspoon of olive oil

Instructions

In a slow cooker, sauté the onion before cooking with the remaining ingredients for 4 to 5 hours.

Honey-Rubbed Pork Wraps

Ingredients

- 12 oz. of boneless pork
- 1 chopped onion
- ½ cup of water
- 2 tablespoons of Worcestershire sauce
- ¼ cup of tomato puree
- 1 teaspoon of garlic ginger paste
- 2 tablespoons of honey
- 1 teaspoon of salt
- Lettuce leaves

Instructions

Apart from the lettuce, mix all ingredients using a slow cooker and leave it on for 11 to 12 hours.

Shrimp & Garlic with Coconut Milk

Ingredients

- 12 oz. of peeled shrimp
- 1 tablespoon of olive oil
- 4 garlic cloves
- ¾ cup of coconut milk
- 1 teaspoon of lemon juice
- Coriander leaves
- 1 teaspoon of salt

Instructions

Sauté olive oil with garlic in a slow cooker. After that, cook the remaining ingredients with the mixture for another five hours.

Mushroom and Chicken Stew

Ingredients

- 1 lb. of chicken breasts
- ½ cup of button mushrooms
- 2 sliced celery stalks
- 1 teaspoon of salt
- ¼ cup of red wine
- 2 garlic cloves
- ½ cup of tomato puree

Instructions

Mix all ingredients within a slow cooker, then cook for about six hours before serving.

Pork Stew and Apple Cider Vinegar

Ingredients

- 1 lb. of pork roast
- 2 tablespoons of apple cider vinegar
- ½ cup of sweet potato
- 1 teaspoon of thyme

- 1 teaspoon of parsley
- 1 teaspoon of salt
- 1 cup of water

Instructions

Mix all ingredients carefully, then transfer the mixture to another slow cooker. Put the lid on and wait for about eleven hours before serving.

Sour and Sweet Pork

Ingredients

- 4 pork chops
- 1½ cups of diced carrots
- 1½ cups of broccoli florets
- 10 oz. of chopped pineapple
- 1 bell pepper
- 2½ tablespoons of Worcestershire sauce
- 2 tablespoons of vinegar
- ½ teaspoon of salt

Instructions

Apart from pineapple, add all ingredients into a big pot and cover the lid. Leave the stove on for at least 7 hours, then add the pineapples. Let the mixture cool down before serving.

Piquant Chicken

Ingredients

- 1 lb. of chopped chicken
- 1 chopped onion
- 2 garlic cloves
- 1½ tablespoons of curry powder
- 1 teaspoon of apple cider vinegar
- 6 raisins
- 5 almonds
- ½ cup of tomato puree

Instructions

Sauté the bell peppers and onions within a slow cooker, then add other ingredients and cook about 7 hours.

IV. CHAPTER III. HIIT – THE ULTIMATE ANTI-DIABETES WEAPON

What Exactly is HIIT?

HIIT is the abbreviation for High Intensity Interval Training. Besides, HITT is sometimes called Sprint Interval Training (SIT) or High Intensity Intermittent Exercise (HIIE). To be specific, HIIT is an improved and revised kind of interval training. Generally, HIIT is defined as an exercise program that combines short sessions of extreme anaerobic exercise with less forceful recovery phases. In other words, it is regarded as a set of cardiovascular workout sessions.

A typical HIIT session lasts between four and thirty minutes. These short, yet intense periods can help you enhance your athletic capacity, along with the condition.

Uncover the Way HIIT Works

Basically, HIIT requires more active movements of muscle fibers than other different types of exercise, thus reducing the levels of muscle glycogen while leading to a dramatic increase in the insulin sensitivity of post-exercise muscles. In other words, practicing HIIT stimulates the production of insulin.

Every HIIT session contain various intense physical exercise and activities. A common interval usually starts with some warm-up exercises, followed by surprisingly intense exercises which are repeated over and over again. Additionally, the sessions are separated by some exercises that have medium intensity.

The purpose of these medium-level exercises is to allow you to recover from those intense workout periods, plus a HIIT session usually ends with a cooling down interval. When it comes to exercises with high intensity, it is suggested that you spend 100% of your effort while you only need to put in half that amount for those with medium intensity.

The length and frequency of every exercise varies, but it is essential that you need to repeat exercises with high intensity at least three 20-second periods. If you practice with a personal trainer, they will have to calculate the appropriate intensity level of the exercises based on your age, gender, condition and other medical situations.

Types of HIIT Regimens

Even though there are many different versions of HIIT created all over the world, Peter Coe is the person who originally developed HIIT. Here is a summary of the four most common versions of HIIT.

The Peter Coe Protocol

Peter Coe, a well-known athletics coach, applied a specific interval training that required high impact, couple with short recovery periods at the end of the 1970s. This regimen was specially inspired by Woldemar Gerschler's principles and PerOlof Astrand's works. Specifically, Peter Coe used to plan multiple HIIT sessions with the repetitions of 200-meter races, along with the recovery intervals of about 30 seconds among the runs.

The Tabata Regimen

The Tabata Regimen has been renowned for being a brand new HIIT version after thorough research was conducted by Izumi Tabata, a professor and his partners in 1996, involving Olympic speed-skaters. According to the study, attendants carried out an intense set of exercises for approximately 20 seconds, combined with a 10-second interval. This cycle is continuously repeated for about 4 minutes.

This series of exercise was executed via a cycle ergometer, along with some mechanical brakes. Tabata named this regimen the IE1 Protocol. Athletes who applied this technique in the study were thoroughly trained four times per week, followed by a steady-state training once a week. The result is that these athletes could produce the same outcomes as those who undertook steady-state training five times per week.

These days, the Tabata protocol is preferred by thousands of people who practice HIIT to burn fat and reduce the development of diabetes.

The Gibala Protocol

Martin Gibala, a professor at McMaster University, and his partners have conduct lots of research regarding different forms of HIIT exercises. According to a specific study in 2009, participants were required to have a three-minute warm-up session before a 60-minute training of intense exercise, paired with a resting period of nearly 75 seconds. This cycle was then repeated for up to twelve times.

Although the Gibala regimen is extremely daunting and demanding, it is overwhelmingly beneficial for your overall health. Later on, Gibala and his team announced a less intense version of the program in the journal Sports & Exercise. This protocol, instead, was created with the view to providing diabetics and sedentary people a lighter option if they had not practiced doing exercise for quite a long time.

To be specific, the Gibala protocol consists of a three-minute warm-up session, with ten repetitions of 60-second exercises, with the combination of 60-second recovery periods. The cycle ended with a cooling-down interval of about five minutes.

The Timmons Regimen

The third HIIT version that I am going to illustrate in this book originally stems from Jamie Timmons, who is a professor at the University of Loughborough. His protocol consists of a total of three sets of two-minute bike exercises, followed by another cycling session of approximately 20 seconds.

It is essential that you practice three times per week, with each session lasting for nearly 21 minutes. This plan is best suited to enhancing the sensitivity of your body to insulin, as well as burning off the extra amount of fat.

The Reasons HIIT are Widely Applied

The development of HIIT training among those who encounter diabetes is rapidly progressing, and there are two main reasons for this spectacular growth.

First and foremost, since it has multiple different versions, HIIT training can be modified based on the physical abilities and fitness levels of individuals. Moreover, HIIT exercises have been proven to help you burn fat, cut down on your blood sugar, and inhibit the development of various diabetes-related symptoms.

The American College of Sports Medicine has recently stated, "HIIT training protocols can be executed under any exercise mode, including walking, aqua training, elliptical cross-training, cycling, and swimming." Therefore, these HIIT workouts are considered as extremely flexible.

Besides, HIIT training regimens offer participants with unlimited fitness benefits such as continuous endurance exercises, yet in a much shorter time. In fact, HIIT workouts are found to burn off more calories than conventional ones, especially post-workout. Specifically, the post-exercise session is named "EPOC," which is the abbreviation form for excess post-exercise oxygen consumption.

The Connection between HIIT and Diabetes

Surprisingly, one twelfth of the normal population is diagnosed with diabetes. Indeed, this disease has witnessed a rapid increase in its popularity over the last couples of years, demonstrated by the fact that one person passes away every 7 seconds due to this condition.

To prevent this shocking figure from rising, we must address and treat diabetes with appropriate methods, and HIIT is scientifically proven to be one of the most efficient ones. Hence, the next segment focuses on the way HIIT functions to reduce the development of diabetes, especially type II diabetes.

How Can Type II Diabetes Be Prevented By HIIT?

Various scientific studies have concluded that HIIT training lowers the levels of glucose, as well as promote positive improvements when it comes to cardiovascular diseases which are usually found in type II diabetes patients. Firstly, the arduous workouts executed when you go through intense intervals accelerate your heartbeat rate.

As the heart beats faster, a larger amount of blood will be pumped to your essential organs, thus making them obtain more oxygen from the bloodstream. Because of these changes, the metabolism is enhanced, leading to more efficient control of your blood sugar levels. Additionally, intense workout sessions let you strengthen your arterial walls, thus lowering the risk of cardiovascular diseases that are popular in diabetics.

Top Tips for an Effective HIIT Training Program

The sessions which are overwhelmingly intense seem to be the most challenging period for the majority of HIIT attendants because they find it hard to maintain the motivation during the rest of the exercise. Therefore, I want to present some tips on how to refrain from giving up.

1. Start off slowly. It takes time for you to familiarize yourself with this training system since your body cannot execute an extremely intense workout session right from the start, so remind yourself to gradually increase the intensity levels so that you can make sure that your body can tolerate it.

For example, you can start with a short period of cardio exercise, running or cycling of about 15 seconds. You can increase this time based on the tolerance of your body, or when you begin to get used to the idea of constantly moving your body and exercising.

2. Opt for favorite exercises. It is recommended that you select the workouts that you enjoy executing in the interval of intense exercises. The reason why you should never do the opposite is because it is supposed that arduous training will help you burn more calories, but that is not the case.

Choosing an exercise you hate is not a smart approach, as you will not have enough motivation to keep up with the plan. You will easily lose interest in this protocol; thus, it is crucial that you choose to do your favorite kinds of exercise.

3. Fuel your energy. As the intensity of the sessions increase, your body ends up burning off more calories. Although that is your goal, do not forget to notice your body's demands amidst the fat-burning desire.

In addition, skipping meals will not do any good, but your body is likely to be weakened, and it will no longer can execute the exercises needed to trigger your metabolic system and remove fat. Therefore, remember to maintain proper protein and carbohydrate consumption to provide enough energy for your body to exercise.

4. Bring along a timer. It is important that you carefully time every interval within your HIIT training program. This is an indispensable step as it will allow you to identify the time you need to start, stop or move onto another one. Furthermore, it enables you to keep track of your performance, as well as raise awareness of the exercise duration.

If a timer is not brought along, you are more likely to lose track of time, leading you to exercise or rest for a longer interval than you are supposed to do. The common problem found in people who forget to bring a timer is that they cannot recognize when the right time to start the intense session or resting period is, thus destroying the training purpose right from the start.

As a result, bringing along a timer is a crucial step to proceed throughout the plan.

5. Pay attention to your body. Make sure that you always listen to what your body says. Do not push your body beyond its limits, as you will not be able to keep up with the plan for a long time by injuring yourself. Instead, it is essential that you adjust the HIIT sessions in response to your body's needs so that you will feel more comfortable working out.

6. Practice a wide range of exercises. Even though HIIT trainers usually advise you to strictly follow a specific set of exercises during every HIIT session, you can also opt for other alternative exercises. Applying a similar routine over a long time might make you feel bored, thus reducing the motivation that you have in the first place. Hence, if you want to substitute one of the HIIT sessions with cycling or swimming, feel free to do that.

7. Do not go beyond 60 seconds. Even if you think that you have enough endurance to extend the high-intensity interval to more than one minute, it means that you are not using as much effort needed. To put it another way, you should feel totally exhausted after such intervals as this is the sign showing that your lungs and muscles are working.

8. Limit the time for tough exercise to 10 seconds. If you cannot endure the entire 60-second intense interval, then you can try using as much effort as you can in a 10-second session instead. You will have to execute more repeated cycles when you don't put in enough effort, thus extending the time of those exercises. Doing less while working harder can promote better results.

9. Recover efficiently. Make sure that you provide your exhausted muscles with a decent amount of time to recover after intense workout exercises. This is extremely important since your muscles need to recuperate and rest. Additionally, the purpose of these recovery periods is to refill your energy for the next session.

10. Time yourself. This is a crucial step because you will can benefit from the training more efficiently if you carefully time every single interval.

11. Do not eliminate low-intensity intervals. If you feel that you can put up with the highly intensive sessions easily, you still need to maintain the resting periods. These intervals allow you to refill your stamina, as well as burn fat and reduce the level of your blood sugar.

12. Consult a doctor. When you decide to follow a particular protocol, it is highly recommended that you talk to a doctor first. Although these regimens are suited to any person regardless of

conditions and ages, asking for a specialist's opinion is always a smart move before starting the whole plan.

Your doctor might give you some helpful pieces of advice in terms of the intensity and exercises that you should include in your training. What's more, type II diabetes patients might suffer from different complications, which is the reason why they are not allowed to execute HIIT training.

13. Keep track of your heart rate, blood pressure and glucose level. These statistics should be regularly updated both before and after every training period. By doing this, you can get your progress under control, as well as find out whether your overall conditions have been enhanced after HIIT performance.

14. Take important medications. If you are prescribed with any diabetes drugs, there is no reason why you must stop taking them unless the doctor instructs you to do something else. Therefore, if your personal doctor allows you to eliminate medications while performing HIIT, then feel free to do that.

V. CONCLUSION

Eliminating diabetes from your life is the desirable goal of any diabetes patient, and it definitely feels like a burden on your shoulder has been lifted up. You may realize that you have been labeled as a "patient" for so long that the title has become so familiar.

With the introduction of the Vedda-based lifestyle modifications, involving the detailed dietary strategies and the science behind HIIT training, you will sooner or later get rid of this terrible condition. So, diabetes will be a story from the past.

In other words, you will no longer have to encounter test strips, finger pricks, injections, avoiding your favorite foods, and constant worry regarding your health. By following this book, you will be back to your normal self, start living again and do the things that you have dreamed to do. Thank you for making it to the end and thank you so much!

Thank you again!

I hope you enjoyed reading my book!

Finally, if you enjoyed this book, write me an honest review about the book – I truly value your opinion and thoughts and I will incorporate them into my next book.